2 Week Bulletproof Diet

The 2 Week Bulletproof Diet Protocol and Recipes That Will Help You To Shed Fat and Rock A New Smoking Body In No Time

AMARPREET SINGH

THE THOUGHT FLAME
TURNING SPARK INTO FLAME

info@thethoughtflame.com

www.thethoughtflame.com

Table of Contents

Introduction

While I may not be the actual creator of the Bulletproof diet, I can testify to how it works. I am a person who follows the diet religiously and I can personally testify to what recipes taste great and which ones actually don't. With the Bulletproof diet you can have the chance to enjoy diverse meals that not only look incredibly creative, but that are appetizing as well. This creativeness helps it to become much easier to adhere to the diet while still enjoying the ride.

Everything said and done, one thing you simply cannot deny is the fact that we live in a nutrition-stripped world. Sure you may see loads of new varieties of food and delicacies beautifully served on your platter. But that does not count as healthy food for nourishment. The market is full of food that is meant for satisfying the tongue and not the overall well-being. That's because right from the time food is sown , to the way it is harvested and finally cooked and consumed, determines the intrinsic quality of it.

As we have advanced in terms of being "civilized", we have also been exposed to numerous diseases that were not seen earlier times. So the smart choice today is to be aware of the options available to us how we can "bulletproof" ourselves with the help of the "Bulletproof Diet."

I hope that this book will give you a better understanding of the Bulletproof diet as a whole and can help you to reap some of the health benefits that I have been able to enjoy. While I understand that every diet is unique and that every diet has its own set of pros and cons, there are no other diets out there that can compare to the Bulletproof diet.

So, what are you waiting for? Let's get started!

Chapter One: What Is The Bulletproof Diet All About?

The bulletproof diet is similar to the popular Paleo/ caveman diet, which is based upon emulating our ancestors, eating food which can be caught, grown or collected, such as meats, fish, seafood, seeds, nuts, vegetables, fruits and oils.

In contrast the bulletproof diet arose from research into biochemistry and human performance, not just emulating our ancestors. As a result the diet reduces toxic health sapping foods, and replaces them with foods that fuel your body, feed your brain and maximize performance. This inevitably overcomes some of the problems that can arise from long term Paleo dieting.

The food ratios for the Bulletproof Diet are relatively simple. The following food types should be eaten in the suggested quantities when following the simple bulletproof diet (ratios can vary if performing a protein fast version of the diet).

Veggie Sources-make up 20% of your total daily calories and will make up to 6 to 11 daily servings.

Fruit or Starch Sources-make up 5% of your total daily calories and up to 1 daily serving. This is a source that you will usually eat in the evenings.

Oil and Fat Sources-make up 50% to 70% of your total daily calories and up to 5 to 9 of your daily servings.

Protein Sources-make up 20% of your total daily calories and up to 4 to 6 of your daily servings.

Food Categories Of The Bulletproof Diet

The food that you will consume while adhering to the Bulletproof Diet will fall into three separate categories:

1. Bulletproof

2. Suspect

3. Toxic

The whole point of this book is to get you to consume foods that only fall into the Bulletproof category as this will be the healthier alternative for you. Now, let's go in depth to see what foods fall into the three categories and why they fall into these categories.

Bulletproof Rating

In a 1 to 5 star rating, the bulletproof rating would definitely fall into the 5 star category. The rating is based upon how effectively the recipes match the recommended foods and ratios of the diet. Recipes with lower ratings contain less quality "bulletproof" foods but are still allowed on the diet.

Suspect Rating

In a 1 to 5 star rating, the Suspect Rating would fall into the 2 to 3 star rating. This rating is based solely upon what foods certain recipes use such as ingredients that could prove harmful to you in the long run. These types of food are generally not allowed to be consumed while on this diet.

Toxic Rating

In a 1 to 5 star rating, the Toxic Rating would actually not be given a rating at all. The reason behind this is because the foods that fit into this category are not nutritious for you at all. In fact they are more prone to do your body harm then good.

How Does The Bullet Proof Diet Work?

When you first begin to check out the bullet proof diet, the first thing you will most likely run into is the bullet proof diet infographic. This is simply a little pdf template that shows you how the Bulletproof diet works and how, with the right amount of changes, can help make a big difference to your overall health. This template will also show you that there are not a lot of major adjustments to make in order to make this diet work for you. This graphic shows you that there are major differences in the way that Bulletproof is different than what many are used to with the Paleo diet.

What does the Bullet Proof Diet Cover?

1. The types of food you eat

2. The way food is handled before you purchase it

3. The way food is cooked

4. The duration food is cooked

5. The extent to which the food is cooked

6. What dietary supplements you need to take while on this diet

The Bullet Proof Diet ensures that you have only eat the freshest foods to boost your body, your mind, and your overall health. It does not only focus on today's health, but also the future health as well. The Bullet Proof Diet focuses on the body's biology and chemistry of the human body and its needs. The focus on the Bullet Proof Diet is to focus on what nutrients the body needs, and how much it needs of it. It also focuses on how the body best absorbs nutrients from food, and what state the food has to be in for complete digestion and maximum usage of your intake.

Chapter Two: How The Bulletproof Diet Works

The Bulletproof diet is specifically designed to reduce the amount of body fat that you have, mental performance and prevent disease while leaving you satisfied and Energized. In this Diet Plan you are advised to eat only when you are hungry and stop when you're satisfied, snacking is not an option here, so you are advised against it. Also, you are allowed to target 50% to 70% of calories from healthy fats which includes all the good fatty foods, 20% from Vegetables, 20% from protein and 5% from fruit or starch.

For Optimum results you are advised to eat more of oil and Fat with Organic Veggies such as zucchini, lettuce, avocado, asparagus etc. And reduced fruit or starch intake to one to two servings per day in the evenings to avoid your triglycerides getting high.

How The Intermittent Fasting Works

This Diet Plan makes it possible to lose fat easily while increasing mental Focus and energy without craving. In this Plan, You start by consuming a cup of bulletproof coffee in the morning this would help increase your mental focus and increase your work energy for the day. I highly recommend that you eat only the food that is listed in this book as they come with high bulletproof rating to achieve optimum result.

The Bulletproof Protein Fasting Method

This Plan aids in the reduction of inflammation. limit your protein intake to 15-25g for about two to three times a week. This would help cleanse and detox your inner-cells without any record of muscle loss. Also, you should consume a cup of bulletproof coffee to keep you full and energized throughout the day, take low carbs meals and high fats the rest of the day. To achieve optimum result , take the foods listed in our recipes with bulletproof rating from 2-3.

Here in this ultimate bulletproof guide, we have specially prepare some easy and quick mouthwatering recipes that would enable you follow through each and every one of this bulletproof diet plan easily. We've done our research and made sure that the ratio of foods we prepared fall into the bulletproof diet approved foods. So, be rest assured that all our recipes are 100% Bulletproof.

Chapter Three: Common Dieting Myths and The Truth Behind Them

In order for you to lose weight with any diet, your body needs five things: energy for your brain, fuel to help drive your body, nutrients for your body cells, no toxins that are unnecessarily harming your body and feeling satisfied throughout the day. The truth of the matter is that many of these popular "diet" are in fact contributing to the obesity problem rather than helping people to lose weight.

These diets are also responsible for spreading many popular diet myths. In this chapter we will take a look at five of the most popular perpetuated myths from the industry and then we will take a look at the classic Bulletproof take on each of the them.

Myth #1: You Are Not Trying Hard Enough If You Are Not Losing Any Weight

This is one of the myths that tends to cause the most harm as there are many people out there who are struggling with their weight right now are touched by this myth. It is not like these people aren't aware of their states, not when the entire world is shoving it down their throats on a daily basis.

The problem is not that these people aren't aware of the health of their bodies, the problem is that on a daily basis they are losing a battle of will to fight their bodies biological need for food. It also doesn't help that society and doctors don't see this as well. Most doctors and people in society today is misunderstand the power of will and wholeheartedly believe that the secret to weight lose is simply buckling down and say no to eating at all.

What these doctors and other people do not understand that we do not have an endless supply of willpower at hand. It is quite possible to run out of willpower and most of the time the people who are overweight have lost their will power long before they decided to get the help they need.

This phenomenon is known as decision fatigue and it is the main factor behind you choosing poor diet choices and loosing the will power to choose a food that is more satisfying and healthier for you in the long run.

Myth #2 You Are Really Not As Hungry As You Believe That You Are

It is true that hunger not only increases your performance, but it is also known to sap your energy and make you cranky and unproductive. It is also responsible for decreasing the willpower that you have.

To be 100% honest, hunger itself is a giant waste of time. It keeps your attention away from things that are important and is more prone to cause you to make more mistakes than you would normally make.

What the Bulletproof diet does is that it essentially hacks your hunger by balancing the hormones which have control of this basic function such as Leptin and Ghrelin.

We all know that hunger is not something that is easy to ignore. However, it is completely manageable as long as you do not give into your food cravings. By following this diet, you will be able to take control over your natural biology so that your hunger will no longer distract you.

Myth #3: The Only Kind of Diet That Is Healthy Is A Low-Fat Diet

Ever since the 1950's food chemists began creating a variety of different low-fat foods to help fight off heart disease. However, whenever you remove the fat from food, you are left with only two things left: protein and sugar. In order to keep this food intact you will need to replace the fat with something else. Unfortunately most food chemists insisted on using sugar as a replacement instead of something a little healthier.

One of the main causes of people failing any diet they start is simply that they feel tortured by not eating foods that are filling and satisfying. You do not have to suffer like that with the Bulletproof diet as you can give yourself the chance to enjoy satisfying foods that are incredibly delicious.

Fat is one of the primary foundations used with the Bulletproof diet, which can prove incredibly nutritious as long as you use the right kinds of fat sources. These fat sources will leave you feeling highly satisfied and this will help you to stick with this diet in the long run.

Myth #4: If You Eat Fat, You In Turn Will Become Fat

This is one of those myths that make us believe that if we eat fat, we will become fat and sick in return. This is a myth that couldn't be any less true. In fact the opposite happens: the more fat that you consume, the more energy your body will produce more energy, which will help you to burn more fat in the long run.

Thanks to all of the falsified research, fat sources have been given a bad reputation for no apparent reason. Not all fat sources are bad. There are plenty of healthy fat sources out there that are not only great for your health, but that are essential for life itself. By using the right kind of fat sources you can help your body and brain function to its highest capacity, burn more calories, cleanse your body and to build up an essential building block needed to sustain your overall health.

Myth #5: Cutting As Many Calories As You Can Is The Only Way That You Can Lose Weight

If you are the type of person who believes that calories are the reason why people gain weight today rather then consuming fat, they you're going to be surprised. The truth of the matter is that it does not matter how many calories you have. In fact your brain uses up to 25% of the total calories that you take in on a daily basis. With that being said, you can take in as many calories as you want without worrying about getting fat in the process.

While cutting calories may help you to lose a tiny bit of weight there are many more factors that go into helping you shed weight such as the temperature of the room that you are in, how much sleep you get and even how hard your breathe.

The moment that you stop focusing on how many calories you take in on a daily basis, the more you will be able to concentrate on the quality of the food that you eat so that you can give your body the proper nutrition that it needs.

Chapter Four: The Problem With Overcooked and Undercooked Foods and The Truth About How You Make Your Food

Not only is it important to know exactly what you are putting into your mouth on a daily basis, but it is also just as important to know what you are cooking your food in. None of this is as important as it is with the Bulletproof Diet. In this chapter we will go in-depth about the consequences of under cooking your food, the consequences of over cooking your food, but what every day items you should avoid using when cooking your food.

The Effects of Undercooking or Overcooking Your Food

1. Overcooking Your Food

Cooking and overcooking food is one of the main reasons that it loses an abundance of its nutrients. Ideally, the body needs as much of a raw diet as possible. As you cook the food, it loses important nutrients and minerals, which cannot be regained through any process.

If food is overcooked , it can also make the body work harder to get what little nutrients that are left, which can cause untimely fatigue. Severely overcooking foods has been proven to result in cancer after long term exposure, especially if it is cooked to the point of charring.

2. Undercooking Your Food

Another serious issue with nutrition is under cooking foods. Undercooking foods can lead to infections from various bacteria. E-coli and Salmonella cause various issues. These issues can lead to small problems like nausea and vomiting to full hospitalization and the need for expensive medical treatment.

What Is The Preferred Way To Eat?

The preferred way to eat food is as raw as possible. Vegetables and fruit should ideally be served raw, or close to raw. If fruits and vegetables must be cooked, they should only be cooked long enough to create the recipe you desire and not thoroughly cooked.

What NOT To Use To Cook Your Food

What you choose to cook in dramatically changes the effects that your food can have. Because of this, you must carefully evaluate your cookware and the heating selection.

A Microwave

Cooking in a microwave is not recommended, for many reasons. Previous concerns were surrounded by the amount of microwaves that escape through the glass. However, this is not the current concern.

Microwaves over cook food, they also help deplete the nutrition in food, and allow food to sit in its own fat and reabsorb it. Because of this, everything that is cooked in a microwave is not healthy for you. So next time you want to reheat that casserole, do not microwave it, you are better off placing it back in the oven to heat up.

Chatting Grill

Charred meat may sound appealing, and may smell delicious, but do not eat it. Recent studies have shown that charred meat can actually increase the risk of cancer. Charred meat is also lacking essential minerals that your body needs.

Since the meat cooks unevenly in a grill and the cooking process can be unpredictable, you can also have places in the meat that contain bacteria that can make you ill.

Chapter Five: How To Lose Weight on The Bulletproof Diet and Need To Know Supplement Facts

When it comes to losing weight with the Bulletproof Diet, Many people have showed serious results using the Bullet Proof Diet. Many of them are shocked at their own results. Why are they loosing this much weight? Well, it is because the Bullet Proof Diet is a way of life. Partnered with exercise and staying active, the Bullet Proof Diet can help you develop a healthy weight, and help you increase the muscle development.

The Bullet Proof Diet isn't a miracle. It only emphasizes what your body actually needs and avoids most of what your body doesn't need.

The Bullet Proof Diet does not say that you

cannot have the things you want, only that you must eat them in moderation. It also emphasizes that you should not deny yourself something that you enjoy, only that you must monitor how much you eat of it. How is that for a diet? You can still eat the things you love!

The best part of the Bullet Proof Diet is that you don't have to swallow a diet pill every day. The main focus of your diet is what you eat and how you cook it, or not cook it. We all know that raw fruits and vegetables are best for us, and the Bullet Proof Diet focus on just this, something that we already know. No surprises, no extra time spent studying things that you are not sure of. Best of all, no more guessing games.

Why spend hours searching for the diet that is right for you when all you really have to do is eat natural foods in their natural state? Of course, you have to cook some foods, such as meat, but knowing to what extent you need to cook the meat will also help you increase your health, lose weight, and prevent disease or illness in the future.

What To Expect When You Are On The Bulletproof Diet

We all known how difficult it is for our bodies to accept dietary changes. Not only when it comes to a mental standpoint, but also when it comes to your very body adjusting to easier to process foods.

While your body adjusts to dietary changes when it is necessary, such as being on the Bulletproof diet, you may experience normal abdominal discomfort. This means that you may have to make a few extra visits to your bathroom from time to time. Why does this happen? It is because your body is trying to adjust to a much healthier lifestyle and is busy flushing out any excess fats that you have managed to store in your body.

While it may take a while for you body to adjust to these chance, it will certainly help you out in the long run. By sticking this diet you are making the job of the digestive tract much easier and will help it save energy from over digesting all of the harsh foods that you once consumed.

A Little Advice On Supplements

There are many diets today that ignore the importance of using supplements as a part of your daily regimen. However, supplements are extremely important, especially when you are not consuming the healthiest foods for yourself or when those healthy foods are not readily available.

Not only does the food that we eat put us at huge risk of not getting enough of the nutrients that we need, but so does the water we drink too. This is because of the current methods that is used to purify water today. These new methods draw out the important vitamins and minerals that we need instead of leaving them in the water for us to consume.

On top of that not all of the vitamins and minerals that we need can be found in our every day normal food. In order to ensure that we get the right amount of vitamins and minerals on a daily basis, you would need to consume about 30,000 calories a day. If you took in that many calories every day for an entire year, you wouldn't be able to fit through your door.

So, while you are on the Bullet proof diet are there specific vitamins and minerals that you should focus on and that you make sure you get on a daily basis?

The answer is yes. The many vitamins that you should focus on getting are Vitamin D, glucarate, Calcium, Fish Oil and Magnesium. These are the vitamins that are necessary if you want to live a much healthier and happier life. Not only do these vitamins help to increase the ability for your system to digest food, but they will also help to increase the overall health of your internal organs, which include your respiratory system and heart.

To make sure that you cover all of your basis by sticking to a single brand of multi-vitamin. This is not enough to get all of the vitamins and minerals that you need. You will need to take a few extra supplements such as B Vitamins, D Vitamins, etc to ensure that you are getting everything that you need.

Chapter Six: Nutritious Bulletproof Diet Breakfast Recipes

Whether you are looking to enjoy a high performance cup of coffee or whether you are looking to enjoy a satisfying early morning meal, you will find the perfect recipes to make in this chapter.

Morning shows the day! Well for me it is the morning meal that shows and shapes the day! You can blame your depleting level of energies through the day, on the breakfast that you chose in the morning. Most of the convenient food options that you are tempted to use so often are the main culprits. Modernity is defined by stacking the larder with ready-to-eat donuts and quick black coffee to waken you up from slumber. Sure you tend to feel full and woken up then, but as the day progresses these things show their dark side as they only tend to make you feel worse.

Sugar-laden cereals that you have been giving your kids so joyously are something extreme and should be avoided at all costs. Other than that, the frozen sausages and salamis that you smartly take out from your freezer to flaunt that smart mom or a hostess in you are also equally to be blamed. That's because, other than being sure that they taste great, are you aware about the quality of meat used in it?

Knowing how much you love your cuppa, here's the very famous Bulletproof Coffee that would leave you full of much needed energy and vigor for the day. It has grass-fed butter in it. And if that makes you squirm and flinch, believe me I also did the same when I heard about it. But this is what people living in high-altitude regions and harsh weather conditions have as their staple beverage for ensuring high energy all through the day. If you have your doubts about fats that come with butter, then you must know that your body is screaming for healthy fats and this butter provides it with just that.

Original Bulletproof Coffee

This creamy cup of coffee will give you the energy that you need to run your busy chaotic life on a daily basis. You can easily make this your breakfast on the go or enjoy with some low-fat yogurt to kick start your day the right way.

Ingredients:

-2 Cups of Coffee, Hot Brewed and Made With Low-Toxin Beans

-2 Tbsp. of Butter, unsalted and Grass Fed

-2 Tbsp. Coconut Oil

Directions:

1. Brew your coffee mixture as you normally would, but make sure that you use a metal filter if you can.

2. While you coffee is brewing add some hot water into a blender. After your coffee brews pour out the hot water and add your freshly brewed coffee, butter and coconut oil into your blender.

3. Cover your blender and blend your coffee until there is a little layer of foam on the top of your mixture.

4. Pour into serving cups and add a dash of cinnamon, dark chocolate, sweetener or vanilla if you want.

Poached Eggs With Some Sautéed Greens

Poaching eggs is one of the best methods to cook eggs if you want to enjoy a Bulletproof meal. Poaching helps your eggs to retain the important nutrients they naturally have. Feel free to serve this with some fresh and organic green so that you can feel satisfied and full in the morning.

Ingredients:

-2 Tbsp. of Butter, Unsalted and Grass Fed

-Dash of Sea Salt For Taste

-2 Eggs, Poached

-2 Tbsp. of Almonds, Sliced Finely

-2 to 3 Cups of Kale and Collards, Freshly and Washed

Directions:

1. Fill a medium sized pan with about an inch or so of water. Add in your mixed greens to cook over medium heat. Cook your greens until they become tender. Drain your water.

2. Next add in your butter and toss your greens gently until completely covered. Remove your greens from heat.

3. Sprinkle your greens with some salt and nuts and toss again to cover. Top with your poached eggs and serve immediately.

Un-Omelet Bulletproof Diet Style

This is a meal that you can enjoy virtually any time of the day. However, this is a great meal to make early in the morning or as a quick lunch.

Ingredients:

-1 Head of Broccoli, Large In Size, Sliced Into Florets and Finely Chopped

-1 Egg Yolk, Raw

-1 Tbsp. C8 MCT Oil

-1 Tbsp. of Lemon Juice

-Dash of Sea Salt For Taste

-Dash of Rosemary, Fresh and For Taste

Directions:

1. The first thing that you will have to do is steam your vegetables and once they are fully steamed, drain them well.

2. After that you will need to pour some hot water into your blender to preheat it slightly. Once your vegetables are ready remove the hot water from the blender and add in your veggies. Next add in the rest of your ingredients.

3. Allow your vegetables to cook your eggs as you blend them on the lowest setting until you have an extremely creamy sauce.

4. Pour into a serving dish and sprinkle with your herbs and sea salt for taste. Enjoy.

Classic Bulletproof Eggs Benedict

Now you can enjoy a classic twist on a delicious breakfast item any time you want with this delicious recipe.

Ingredients:

-1 Avocado, Ripe

-3 Handfuls of Spinach, Washed and Drained

-Dash of Sea Salt For Taste

-2 Eggs, Softly Poached

-Some Hollandaise Sauce

-1 Tbsp. of Butter, Unsalted and Grass Fed

Directions:

1. Using a medium sized pan, add in your spinach with about 2 Tbsp. of Water. Sauté your spinach until slightly wilted.

2. Then strain the water from your pan and add in your butter and salt. Continue to sauté until the butter is fully melted. Place your spinach onto a serving plate.

3. Place your poached eggs on top of your spinach and drizzle with a touch of hollandaise sauce. Serve with a slice of fresh avocado and enjoy.

Wholesome Baked Grapefruit With A Touch of Cinnamon

There is nothing better to wake up to then a hearty breakfast that contains fresh fruits. With the sweet taste of grapefruit and a touch of cinnamon, this dish will leave you craving more.

Ingredients:

-Dash of Cinnamon, Organic

-Sprinkle of Nuts, Organic and Your Personal Choice

-1 Grapefruit, Medium In Size and Organic

Directions:

1. Slice your grapefruit in half using a serrated knife. Then slowly loosen the sections of the grapefruit as carefully as possible.

2. Next place your grapefruit pieces onto a baking sheet. Make sure that you sprinkle each slice with a generous amount of cinnamon and finely chopped nuts.

3. Set your oven to broil and place your grapefruit slices into the oven. Broil for the

next 4 to 6 minutes or until the tops of the grapefruit slightly brown. Remove from oven and serve immediately.

Filling Early Morning Beef Patties

These beef patties make the perfect addition to a plate of poached eggs. They not only taste amazing, but they will leave you feel extremely full as well.

Ingredients:

-2 Pounds of Beef, Ground and Grass Fed

-1 tsp. of Sea Salt For Taste

-1 Tbsp. of Thyme, Fresh and Organic

-1 Tbsp. of Rosemary, Fresh and Organic

-1 Tbsp. of Coconut Oil, Organic and Extra Virgin

Directions:

1. Preheat your oven to 350 degrees.

2. Then using a large size mixing bowl, combine your beef, freshly ground herbs and dash of sea salt.

3. Using your hands mix your ingredients thoroughly until mixed well. Then form your mixture into thick sized patties.

4. Next, grease a medium sized baking pan with some coconut oil and cook your patties for the next 25 to 30 minutes or until they are thoroughly cooked through.

Early Morning Breakfast Salad

Who said a wholesome salad is only something that can be enjoyed for lunch only? With this delicious recipe you can enjoy a hearty salad right before you head out to work.

Ingredients:

-1 Carrot Stick, Fresh and Organic

-1 Celery Stick, Fresh and Organic

-2 Eggs, Large In Size and Pastured

-5 Ounces of Baby Spinach, Fresh and Organic

-Dash of Sea Salt For Taste

-A Small Dab of Coconut Oil, Extra Virgin

-1 Avocado, Ripe and Organic

-1 Broccoli Floret, Fresh and Organic

Directions:

1. Using a vegetable peeler to remove the carrot peelings on the carrot. Then, cut your carrot into tiny pieces and place the pieces into a large sized salad bowl.

2. Next, cut up your celery and place it in the salad bowl. Then, remove the central part of

the avocado, slice it up into small sized pieces. Next place the avocado into the salad bowl as well.

3. Next dice up your baby spinach and broccoli. Place your broccoli into a pot of boiling water and boil your broccoli for about 5 to 7 minutes. Then add in your spinach and boil it until it wilts. This should take about 2 to 3 minutes. Remove from pot and set aside to cool.

4. Once fully cooled, place both your boiled spinach and broccoli into your salad bowl along with your other vegetables.

5. Then prepare your eggs in any way that you like using your coconut oil.

6. Top your salad with your eggs and season with your dash of sea salt. Toss gently and serve immediately. Enjoy.

Savory Egg Muffins

Muffins are perhaps the easiest breakfast items that you can make. Not only do they take little to no time at all to prepare, but they are the perfect breakfast items to make if you are looking to enjoy a tasty breakfast meal on the go.

Ingredients:

-Dash of Sea

-¼ Cup of Cilantro, Organic, Fresh and Finely Chopped

-¼ Cup of Green Onions, Fresh, Organic and Finely Chopped

-Dab of Coconut Oil, Organic and Extra Virgin

-12 Eggs, Large In Size and Pastured

Directions:

1. Preheat your oven to 350 degrees. While it

heats up lightly grease a muffin tin with a generous amount of oil or butter.

2. Next chop up your cilantro and onions. Set aside.

3. Whisk your eggs using a large sized mixing bowl and add in your sea salt.

4. Then stir in your cilantro and onion mixture. Mix your muffin batter until thoroughly combined and pour into your muffin tins.

5. Place into your oven to bake for the next 20 to 25 minutes or until the eggs are fully set.

Fruity Health Bars

If you are looking for healthy breakfast bars that you can easily take along with you, then this is the perfect recipe for you. These are relatively simple to make and taste incredible.

Ingredients:

-½ tsp. of Sea Salt, For Taste

-3 Cups of Assorted Nuts, Of Your Choice and Organic

-1 Cup of Cranberries, Dried and Organic

-½ Cup of Honey, Raw

-¼ Cup of Coconut Oil, Extra Virgin and Organic

-1 tsp. of Cinnamon, Ground and Organic

-2 Cups of Shredded Coconut, Unsweetened and Organic

Directions:

1. Place some parchment paper into a medium sized baking dish and set aside.

2. Then pour your assorted nuts into a large sized mixing bowl and combine thoroughly.

3. Next take one cup of your assorted nut mixture out of your bowl and place them onto a medium sized cutting board. Chop up your nuts into fine pieces.

4. Then take your remaining two cups of assorted nuts and place them into a blender or food processor. Pulse the nuts until they are chopped to a small enough size that they can be put into your fruit bars.

5. Then, add all of your nuts from both your food processor and cutting board back into your mixing bowl. Toss with your hands to thoroughly combine.

6. Next add in your dried cranberries and shredded coconut to your mixing bowl. Stir thoroughly to combine your mixture until mixed well.

7. Using a small sized saucepan add your coconut oil, cinnamon, sea salt, and honey.

Cook your mixture over medium to low heat, making sure that you stir until your mixture begins to bubble slightly. Once your mixture begins to bubble remove it from heat.

8. Next pour your liquid over your nut mixture in your mixing bowl. Stir thoroughly to combine until everything is evenly mixed.

9. Once mixed well pour all of your ingredients into your baking dish.

10. Then use a second sheet of parchment paper and firmly press it over your mixture until it is well packed together. Let your mixture sit for about two hours. Then, cover and place into your freezer to freeze for at least one or two hours.

11. Then use your parchment paper to take the granola mixture out of your baking dish as gently as possible. Transfer your granola onto a small sized cutting board. Next using a sharp

knife, slice your granola into thin bars. Set aside and save your granola for whenever you are ready to enjoy them.

Filling Scrambled Eggs With A Side of Asparagus

Who doesn't enjoy bacon in the morning? Well, for all of you bacon lovers out there, this recipe is specially designed for you. Not only does it taste amazing, but it is incredibly nutritious as well.

Ingredients:

-4 Strips of Bacon Fat, Pastured

-1 ½ Cups of Bell Pepper, Any Color, Fresh, Peeled, Deseeded and Finely Diced

-4 Eggs, Large In Size and Pastured

-1 Tomato, Medium In Size and Diced Finely

-¼ Cup of Spinach, Baby, Fresh and Packed Lightly

-1 Onion, Medium In Size, White and Diced Finely

-Dash of Sea Salt and Pepper For Taste

Directions:

1. Preheat your oven to 350 degrees.

2. While your oven heats up use a medium sized skillet or sauce pan, start cooking your bacon strips over medium heat. Be careful that you don't crisp them. Make sure that you leave them a little raw.

3. Next add in your diced onions, tomatoes and peppers and sauté them in the pan with the bacon for at least 7 minutes or until they start to cook through. Set aside.

4. Then take out a medium sized bowl and crack your eggs into it. Beat them lightly and

season them with your salt and pepper.

5. Then take a cup cake baking tray and line the cups with silicone baking cups. Spoon your bacon and vegetable mixture in each cup, making sure to fill each cup halfway.

6. Next take your bowl with the eggs and pour the beaten eggs on top until the cups are almost full.

7. Place them into your oven to bake for at least 17 minutes in the oven or until the eggs are set. Remove from oven.

8. Take out one cupcake sized omelet and serve immediately. Enjoy.

Chapter Seven: Delicious Bulletproof Lunch and Dinner Recipes

If you are looking for a highly nutritious and filling lunch or dinner recipe, this is the chapter for you. In this section you will only find the healthiest entrees that follow the Bulletproof protocol.

One thing that Bulletproof Diet stresses upon is the consumption of grass-fed meat and not grain -fed one. For this you really need to get picky about the meat you buy. You must ensure where it is from. The same holds true for fish and sea food as well. Just quit the regular cans of tuna that you have been used to of buying from the supermarket. These are not just laden with preservatives at the time of packaging but also come with high level of exposure to general environmental pollution. Wild caught sea food is what is recommended best for the Bulletproof Diet program. And if you love your daily dose of meat, these are the recipes for you.

Savory Chicken and Vegetable Soup

This is the perfect soup recipe for you to warm you up on the cold weekend nights. It is filling, nutritious and incredibly easy to make.

Ingredients:

-4 Cups of Water, Warm

-1 Clove of Garlic, Minced

-1 Onion, Medium In Size and Diced Finely

-1 Cup of Chicken, Whole, Pastured and Finely Diced

-1 Zucchini, Small In Size, Peeled and Diced Finely

-2 Carrots, Diced Finely

-4 Tomatoes, Medium In Size and Medium

-1 Bay Leaf

-Dash of Sea Salt and Pepper For Taste

Directions:

1. Take a large pot and on medium heat, combine the water, chicken, onion, bay leaf, pepper and garlic.

2. Allow the water to come to a boil. Turn the heat down. Place a cover on top of the pot and let it simmer for 2 hours or until the chicken becomes tender. Uncover the pot and remove the bay leaf.

3. Now add the remaining ingredients and allow the soup to come to a boil again before reducing the heat again.

4. Place a cover on top and let the soup simmer for 20 minutes more or until the vegetable are tender. Serve hot with some steamed vegetables on the side or have as is.

Tasty Pastured Chicken Legs

This is the perfect recipe to make to go along with a tasty salad or can be enjoyed simply by itself. Easy to make and incredibly healthy.

Ingredients:

-Dash of Sea Salt and Pepper For Taste

-4 Chicken Legs, Pastured and Just Thighs

-1 tsp. of Cayenne Pepper

-½ Cup of Almond Meal

-1 tsp. of Mustard, Dry

-1 tsp. of Curry Powder

-4 Tbsp. of Olive Oil

Directions:

1. Leave your oven to preheat at 350 degree. While your oven heats up, take a baking dish and line it with some baking paper and set aside.

2. Take a large bowl and add the almond meal, curry powder, cayenne, dry mustard and some salt and pepper. Mix them well and then set aside.

3. Clean the chicken thighs and quarters and rub each piece generously with olive oil. Crumb each thigh by rolling it in the almond meal mix you made. Make sure they are all coated well and give each one a light shake to remove excess almond meal.

4. Place them on the baking paper and pop the dish in the oven. Cook for an hour or until the coating gets crispy.

5. Test the chicken by piercing them with a skewer. If the juices run clear, take them out, otherwise, cook for 10 minutes more then check again.

6. Serve either by itself or with a side of steamed vegetables and enjoy.

California Style Sweet Potatoes and Kale

This is a perfect recipe for you during your intermittent fasting phase of this protocol. It will help to curb your cravings while still fueling your body with the energy that it needs.

Ingredients:

-5 Sweet Potatoes, Chopped Finely

-1 Cauliflower, Large In Size, Cut Into Small Cubes

-3 Onions, Small In Size and Chopped Finely

-1 Cup of Kale, Fresh and Finely Chopped

-4 Bell Peppers, Fresh and Finely Chopped

-1 Cup of Coconut Oil

-1 tsp. of Coriander, Ground

-1 Tbsp. of Cumin, Ground

-3 Squeezes of Lemon Juice, Fresh

-Dash of Sea Salt and Pepper For Taste

-3 Tbsp. of Water, Warm

-4 Avocados, Ripe and Finely Sliced

Directions:

1. Preheat your oven to 350 degrees. After your oven heats up place your potatoes into your oven and allow to bake for 30 minutes or until they become tender.

2. Then take a large pot and heat oil in it. Add in your bell pepper, onions, salt and black pepper.

3. Next, add in your kale and cook until all of the ingredients become tender. Then add in your cauliflower and water. Allow to cook with the lid on for the next 20 minutes.

4. Last add in your baked potatoes and squeeze lime juice on top. Let it simmer for 10 minutes and then serve.

Filling Kale Salad With A Side of Avocado

This is a great recipe to put together especially if you are looking to make something that is not only filling, but one of the healthiest dishes that you can make.

Ingredients:

-½ Of A Cucumber, Sliced Finely

-½ Of A Head of Kale, Fresh and Torn

-1 Avocado, Fresh

-1 Handful of Almonds, Fresh

-½ Of A Lemon, Used For Fresh Juice

-Dash of Sea Salt For Taste

-1 Handful of Radishes, Finely Sliced

Directions:

1. Toss your kale and avocado together, using your hands until well mixed.

2. Then add in your radishes, cucumbers, and almonds.

3. Finally toss your salad with some fresh lemon juice and sea salt until thoroughly coated and serve at once.

Caribbean Style Chicken

This recipe will give a classic dish and unique and zesty taste. This is a great dish to serve with a fresh bowl of steamed veggies or a simple healthy salad.

Ingredients:

-2 Ounces of Rum, Your Favorite Brand

-1 ½ Tbsp. of Lime Juice, Fresh

-1 Tbsp. of Brown Sugar, Packed

-½ tsp. of Cinnamon, Ground

-¼ tsp. of Cayenne Pepper

-¼ tsp. of Cloves, Ground

-½ tsp. of Ginger, Ground

-1 tsp. of Black Pepper, For Taste

-½ tsp. of Sea Salt, For Taste

-1 Tbsp. of Vegetable Oil

-3 Pounds of Chicken, Pastured

Directions:

1. Preheat your oven to 325 degrees. While it heats up use a small sized mixing bowl and combine your fresh lime juice, rum and brown sugar together until thoroughly mixed. Set aside.

2. Next mix together your cayenne pepper, fresh cloves, ground cinnamon, ground ginger, dash of pepper and dash of sea salt in a separate bowl. Toss together until mixed well.

3. Then brush your chicken with some oil, then coat it with your spice mixture.

4. Then place your chicken into a roasting pan, and bake for about 90 minutes, or until the juices run clear or until a meat thermometer reads 180 degrees.

5. Next, baste your chicken with its own sauce every 20 minutes while it's cooking. Allow the chicken to rest for about 10 minutes before carving it.

Bulletproof Style Meatloaf

Who says that you can't enjoy meatloaf, even if it is done bulletproof style? This meatloaf recipe will surely impress all of your guests and will leave them wanting more.

Ingredients:

-2 Eggs, Large In Size and Pastured

-1 Pound of Beef, Grass Fed

-1 Onion, Medium In Size, Red and Chopped Finely

-2 Cloves of Garlic, Minced

-¼ Cup of Cilantro, Fresh and Finely Chopped

-½ Cup of Parsley, Fresh and Finely Chopped

-½ Of A Red Pepper, Peeled, Deseeded and Finely Chopped

-Dash of Sea Salt and Pepper For Taste

-1 tsp. of Cumin, Powder

-1 Tbsp. of Coconut Oil

Directions:

1. Leave your oven to preheat at 350 degrees. While it heats up take out a baking dish and line it with some baking paper (parchment paper) and set aside.

2. Next take out a large sized bowl and add all of your ingredients, including the pastured eggs, onion, ground beef, the herbs and garlic and cumin powder. Season with your dash of salt and pepper and mix together until combined well.

3. Once everything is evenly combined, take out the baking tray you prepared earlier and place your mixture into it.

4. Then pop it into your oven and cook for the 45 minutes or until the meatloaf starts turning golden brown in color.

5. Then use a skewer to pierce and test the center of the meatloaf. If it isn't fully cooked, bake for an additional 10 minutes.

6. Serve with a light salad or bowl of steamed vegetables and enjoy thoroughly.

Tasty Pineapple Chicken

This recipes will give you the zest and sweetness that you have been looking for. This is a great recipe to make if your are planning a dinner party and are looking for a dish to "wow" your guests.

Ingredients:

-1 Tomato, Medium In Size, Fresh and Finely Sliced

-3 Chicken Breasts, Pastured

-4 Pineapple Rings

-2 Tbsp. of Lime Juice, Fresh

-Dash of Sea Salt and Pepper For Taste

-4 Tbsp. of Water, Warm

-4 Tbsp. of Olive Oil

Directions:

1. Heat up some oil in medium sized skillet and cook until completely browned.

2. Sprinkle your sea salt, pepper and water into the skillet. Allow to cook with the lid on for about 10 minutes.

3. Once the steam begins to cook your chicken, allow it to continue cooking until the steam makes it soft.

4. Next, grill your pineapples on your grill and then add to chicken to the grill.

5. Add in your lime juice, tomato slices and allow to cook for about 10-15 minutes at medium heat until fully cooked through.

6. Serve immediately and enjoy.

Savory Beef Stew

This is the perfect dish to make during the cold winter months. Not only will it leave you feeling warm, but it will leave you feeling satisfied and craving more.

Ingredients:

-6 Cups of Water, Warm

-12 Ounces of Beef, Grass Fed and Cut Into Cubes

-1 Cup of Sweet Potatoes, Sliced Into Cubes

-2 Onions, Large In Size and Diced Finely

-1 Can of Tomatoes, Sliced Into Cubes

-½ Cup of Olive Oil

-2 Red Bell Peppers, Fresh and Finely Diced

-4 Cloves of Garlic, Minced

-4 tsp. of Lemon Juice, Fresh

-2 tsp. of Red Chili Powder

-Dash of Sea Salt and Pepper For Taste

-Some Paleo Bread, To Be Used For Serving and Dipping

Directions:

1. Heat up your oil in a crock-pot and add in your beef, diced potatoes, sliced tomatoes,

sliced onions, fresh bell peppers, warm water, minced garlic, chili powder, fresh lemon juice, dash of salt and dash of pepper.

2. Cook on the highest setting for the next 40 minutes or until a thick gravy begins to form.

3. Serve with your fresh paleo bread and enjoy.

Fresh Sesame Seed Green Beans

This is a delicious and healthy dish that you can serve alongside a fresh salad or other entrée. It is light on your belly, but still will give your body the fuel it needs.

Ingredients:

-½ Cup of Water, Warm

-¾ Pound of Green Beans, Fresh

-1 Tbsp. of Soy Sauce

-2 tsp. of Sesame Seeds, Fresh and Toasted

-1 Tbsp. of Almond Butter

Directions:

1. In a medium sized saucepan, bring your green beans and water together to a rolling boil. Then reduce the heat to medium.

2. Cover and allow the beans to cook until they are crisp and tender. This should take about 10-15 minutes. Once done, drain completely.

3. Next add in your soy sauce, almond butter, and sesame seeds. Toss gently to evenly coat the green beans and serve at once.

Classic Beef Stir Fry With Veggies

If you are looking to spice up your dinner or lunch menu, this is the perfect recipe for you. With this recipe you can enjoy a classic Asian dish with a healthy bulletproof spin on it.

Ingredients:

-1 Clove of Garlic, Pressed

-12 Ounces of Sirloin Steak, Trimmed, Boneless and Thinly Sliced

-2 Tbsp. of Olive Oil

-1 Onion, Yellow, Medium In Size and Thinly Sliced

-2 Stalks of Celery, Chopped Finely

-1 Red Bell Pepper, Deseeded and Cut Into Thin Strips

-¼ Cup of Wine, Burgundy

-3 Tbsp. of Lemon Juice

-Dash of Sea Salt and Pepper For Taste

-4 Ounces of Carrots, Thinly Sliced

-4 Ounces of Mushrooms, Thinly Sliced

Directions:

1. Take a large skillet and on medium heat, add the garlic, half of the wine and a tablespoon of oil. Sauté the beef for 5 to 7 minutes or until the beef starts browning. Scoop out the beef and set aside. Heat some more olive oil and sauté the red pepper, celery, carrots and onion for 4 minutes or until the onion becomes tender. Add the remaining wine, mushrooms and lemon juice to the skillet. Stir-fry all the vegetables together for 3more minutes. Add the meat and stir-fry for another minute more before taking it off the heat.

Roasted Chestnuts With Paleo Style Coconut Macaroons

This recipe is specifically for the protein fasting method. Not only will it help you to lose weight, but it is low in fat and incredibly tasty as well.

Ingredients:

-2 Eggs, Whites Only and Pastured

-1 tsp. of Vanilla

-½ Cup of Honey, Raw

-2 Tbsp. of Coconut Oil

-Dash of Sea Salt For Taste

-1 Lemon, Zest Only

-1 tsp. of Vanilla Extract

-1 ½ Cup of Coconut, Grated

Ingredients For The Coating:

-1 tsp. of Coconut Oil

-1 Tbsp. of Chestnuts, Roasted

-3 ½ Ounces of Chocolate, Dark

Directions:

1. Preheat your oven at 350 degrees. While it

heats up take out a baking dish and line it with some baking paper. and set aside.

2. Then using a large sized bowl, combine your honey, lemon zest, vanilla, sea salt and the egg whites together using a whisk until all of the ingredients are evenly mixed together. Keep whisking until it becomes foamy.

3. Next add in your coconut oil and the coconut flakes into your bowl. Whisk again until thoroughly combined. Set aside and let your mixture rest for about 20 minutes.

4. Then take a tablespoon and use it to tightly pack a ball of the mixture. Place your ball onto your baking sheet. Continue making the balls of mixture until all of your batter has been used up.

5. Place your baking sheet into your oven and allow it to bake for about 10 to 12 minutes or until the macaroons begin to turn gold in color.

6. Remove from your oven and transfer them onto a wire rack to cool.

7. Then use a double broiler and melt your dark chocolate. Then mix it together with your coconut oil in a small sized bowl.

8. Once the coconut macaroons have cooled completely, dip one end into your chocolate while the chocolate is still piping hot. Then sprinkle some of your chestnuts on top and allow the chocolate cool.

9. Serve with a side of coconut cream and enjoy when you are ready.

Fresh Buttered Scallops

This is another great recipe to try during your bulletproof protein fasting phase. This is an easy recipe to put together and is a great one to make if you are looking to impress a few people at a dinner party.

Ingredients:

-2 tsp. of Ginger, Paste and Fresh

-2 Tbsp. of Coconut Oil

-2 tsp. of Garlic, Paste and Fresh

-½ Cup of Shallots, Fresh and Minced

-¼ tsp. of Cumin, Ground

-¼ Cup of Tomato Paste

-¼ tsp. of Cinnamon, Ground

-1 ½ tsp. of Garam Masala

-8 Ounces of Coconut Cream

-1 Pound of Scallops, Sea, Fresh and Cleaned

-Dash of Sea Salt, For Taste

-Dash of Pepper For Taste

-Dash of Cayenne Pepper For Taste

-Dash of Cilantro, Fresh and For Garnish

Directions:

1. Take out a large wok and heat up your coconut oil over medium to high heat.

2. Then add in your shallots and allow to cook for about 2 to 3 minutes or until the shallots begin to soften.

3. Next add in your tomato paste, ginger paste, garlic paste, garam masala, cumin, cayenne, cinnamon and season with salt and pepper. Stir thoroughly to combine all of the ingredients together. All to cook for an additional 3 to 5 minutes, constantly stirring the entire time.

4. Add in your fresh scallops and your coconut cream to the pan and stir to combine everything. Cook for another 5 minutes or until the scallops are fully cooked through.

5. Remove from heat and sprinkle your fresh

cilantro on top of it all. Serve while still piping hot.

Creamy Tomato Soup

This recipe is an excellent one to put together especially during those cold fall and winter nights. This recipe is extremely creamy and will leave you begging for more.

Ingredients:

-½ Cup of Tomatoes, Fresh and Diced

-2 Tbsp. of Olive Oil

-2 tsp. of Garlic, Minced

-1 Cup of Tomato Paste

-2 Liters of Chicken Stock, Pastured

-3 tsp. of Basil, Dried

-½ tsp. of Marjoram, Dried

-1 Bay Leaf

-1/3 tsp. of Thyme, Dried

-½ tsp. of Oregano, Dried

-Dash of Sea Salt and Pepper For Taste

Directions:

1. Using a large sized skillet, sauté your onions over medium to high heat until the onions begin to turn translucent.

2. Then add in your garlic, tomatoes paste and cook for an additional 5 minutes.

3. Next add in your chicken stock , marjoram, thyme, basil, oregano, bay leaf and diced tomatoes. Bring this mixture to a rolling boil and then cook for an additional 30 minutes at low heat. Cover and let simmer.

4. Once fully cooked serve and enjoy while it is still piping hot.

Savory Beef Bake With Zucchini

This grass fed recipe is another great recipe to put together during the protein fasting phase. It is incredibly filling and the zucchini is incredibly tender, making a meal that will soon become a favorite in your household.

Ingredients:

-¼ tsp. of Pepper

-½ tsp. of Oregano, Dried

-1 Pound of Beef, Ground and Grass Fed

-1 Cup of Onion, Finely Chopped

-1 Cup of Celery, Finely Chopped

-4 Zucchini, Sliced Into ¼ inch Slices

-Some Olive Oil

-1 tsp. of Salt

-1, 6 Ounce Can of Tomato Paste

-1 Cup of Mushrooms, Finely Sliced

-2 Cups of Mozzarella Cheese, Shredded

Directions:

1. Preheat your oven to 350 degrees. While your oven heats up place your zucchini onto a baking dish and arrange so that none of the zucchini are touching.

2. Then using a small sized skillet add in your onion, celery and oil. Sauté over medium to high heat for the next 5 minutes or until the onions begin to turn translucent.

3. Then add in your ground beef and cook until it is fully browned. Place you zucchini into the oven and allow to cook until the zucchini is fully tender. Remove from oven.

4. Pour your zucchini into your skillet and mix thoroughly with your ground beef mixture. Remove from heat and serve immediately.

A Traditional Mexican Meal

If you are looking to put together a perfect meal for a classic Mexican night, this is certainly the dish for you. With this dish you will get a little bit of spiciness and a little bit of a tangy flavor.

Ingredients:

-1/3 Cup of Cheddar Cheese, Shredded

-¼ Cup of Salsa, Chunky and Fresh

-4 Eggs, Large In Size, Pastured and Poached

-2 Tbsp. of Sour Cream

-2 Tbsp. of Cilantro, Fresh and Finely Chopped

-2 Tbsp. of Olives, Fresh and Finely Sliced

-1/3 Cup of Avocado, Fresh and Sliced Into Chunks

Directions:

1. Cook your 4 eggs by poaching them and set

aside once they are done.

2. Next heat up your salsa in microwave or on your stovetop over medium to high heat.

3. Then place your poached eggs onto a medium sized serving plate and top with your salsa, sour cream, olives, avocado, parsley and cheese.

4. Serve immediately and enjoy.

Chapter Eight: 2 Week Bulletproof Meal Plan

Now that you understand how the Bulletproof Diet works and how it will help you to lose weight, it is time to set you up on a two week meal plan to help put everything you have learned into practice.

Each of the meals in this 2 week meal plan can be found in this book so feel free to use the recipes given or feel free to use whatever other Bulletproof recipes that you may find.

Day 1

Breakfast

1. Bulletproof Coffee

2. 1 Cup of Fresh Fruit, Your Choice of Fruit

Lunch

1. Savory Chicken and Veggie Soup

Dinner

1. 1 Cup of Steamed Veggies

2. Healthy Kale Salad

Day 2

Breakfast

1. Poached Eggs with Sautéed Greens

Lunch

1. 1 Cup of Steamed Veggies

2. Savory Beef Stew

Dinner

1. Savory Tomato Soup

2. 1 Cup of Steamed Veggies

Day 3

Breakfast

1. 1 Cup of Bulletproof Coffee

2. 1 Cup of Fresh Fruit, Your Choice of Fruit

Lunch

1. Filling Chicken Legs

Dinner

1. 1 Cup of Steamed Veggies or Bulletproof Friendly Baguette

2. Savory Beef Stew

Day 4

Breakfast

1. 1 Cup of Fresh Fruit, Your Favorite Fruit

2. Classic Eggs Benedict

Lunch

1. Sesame Seed Green Beans

Dinner

1. Classic Beef Stir Fry With Veggies

Day 5

Breakfast

1. Bulletproof Style Coffee

2. 1 Cup of Fresh Fruit

Lunch

1. Bulletproof Style Meatloaf

Dinner

1. 1 Cup of Steamed Veggies

2. Pineapple Chicken Dinner

Day 6

Breakfast

1. Bulletproof Coffee

2. Early Morning Breakfast Salad

Lunch

1. Roasted Chestnuts

2. 1 Cup of Steamed Veggies

Dinner

1. Traditional Mexican Meal

Day 7

Breakfast

1. 1 Cup of Fresh Fruit, Your Favorite Kind

2. Early Morning Breakfast Patties

Lunch

1. Bulletproof Coffee

Dinner

1. Beef Bake With Zucchini

Day 8

Breakfast

1. Un-Omelet

2. Bowl of Fresh Fruit, Your Favorite Kind

Lunch

1. Kale with Sweet Potatoes

Dinner

1. Creamy Tomato Soup

2. 1 Cup of Steamed Veggies

Day 9

Breakfast

1. Scrambled Eggs With Asparagus

Lunch

1. Roasted Chestnuts

Dinner

1. Savory Beef Stew

Day 10

Breakfast

1. Bulletproof Coffee

2. 2 Health Bars

Lunch

1. Healthy Kale Salad

Dinner

1. 1 Cup of Steamed Veggies

2. Savory Beef Stir Fry

Day 11

Breakfast

1. Egg Muffins

2. 1 Bowl of Fresh Fruit, Your Favorite Kind

Lunch

1. Caribbean Style Chicken

Dinner

1. Chicken Legs

Day 12

Breakfast

1. Bulletproof Coffee

2. 1 Bowl of Fresh Fruit, Your Favorite Kind

Lunch

1. Traditional Beef Bake with Zucchini

Dinner

1. Chicken and Veggie Soup

Day 13

Breakfast

1. Bulletproof Coffee

2. Classic Eggs Benedict

Lunch

1. 1 Bowl of Steamed Veggies

2. Kale Salad with Avocado

Dinner

1. Traditional Meatloaf

Day 14

Breakfast

1. 1 Bowl of Fresh Fruit

2. Bulletproof Coffee

Lunch

1. 2 Health Bars

Dinner

1. 1 Cup of Steamed Veggies

2. Kale With Sweet Potatoes

By following this Bulletproof Meal Plan to the T you will give yourself the best chance to lose the weight you want, while still maintaining a healthy diet. After 14 days feel free to continue with the diet plan to maximize results for as long as you want. The longer you follow the Bulletproof Diet Protocol, the healthier you will be in the long run.

Conclusion

To lose weight is very easy if you know the process and how to go about it. That is the reason for this Book, to help you achieve your weight loss goal in No time. Get in shape while eating the foods you love. Take advantage of this healthy and delicious recipes provided for you in this book to maximize the results that you are looking for.

For many, "Bulletproof Diet" has been an eye-opener and they have been happy to include it as a part of everyday diet and way of life . Incorporate in this book, you would find all recipes that would help you find your lost energy and vigor. Once you have attuned yourself to this amazing way of preparing and also enjoying your food, there is no looking back. You are right on the road to great health and happiness all the way!

Remember, the only bad actions that you can ever take is by making no action at all. Take the step to a healthier future today by utilizing the diet plan, tips and recipes in this eBook.

About Us

The Thought Flame is committed to add value to its customers through various books, online courses and other resources. You can learn more about us and our books at www.thethoughtflame.com.

Don't forget to check out our amazing **online video courses** at www.thethoughtflame.com/courses/ to take your knowledge to another level.

To check out our **extraordinary collection of diet/cookbooks**, visit http://www.thethoughtflame.com/category/non-fictional/cookbooks/ .

As a part of our valued relationship with our customers, we keep providing you free promotional books, courses and other stuff on subscribing with us on our site. We have a strict anti-spam policy and assure you no spam mails will be sent to your mailbox.

To subscribe with us, visit www.thethoughtflame.com.

Like our work and would like to say thanks?

Buy us a cup of coffee at www.thethoughtflame.com/coffee/

Author

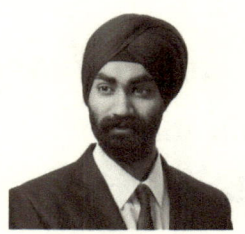

Amarpreet Singh is an avid learner and his passion for education has made him travel, work and study all across the world. He holds three masters degrees, including MBA, from top universities in Asia.

He is author of dozens of books, many of which are Amazon's bestseller, varying in various topics and categories. He also teaches many online courses having thousands of students across the world.

He has a keen interest in international affairs, economics, global poverty and politics, financial markets and entrepreneurship, and strives to be part of a community that shares the same passion.

He has worked as consultant with organizations like Airbus and The World Bank. He loves travelling and learning about new cultures, and has been fortunate to live/work/travel/study in countries like India, China, Korea, US, South Africa, Japan, Philippines, Singapore, Canada etc., and learn about the culture and lifestyle in each of them. To check out more of his work, visit www.thethoughtflame.com